AF594383

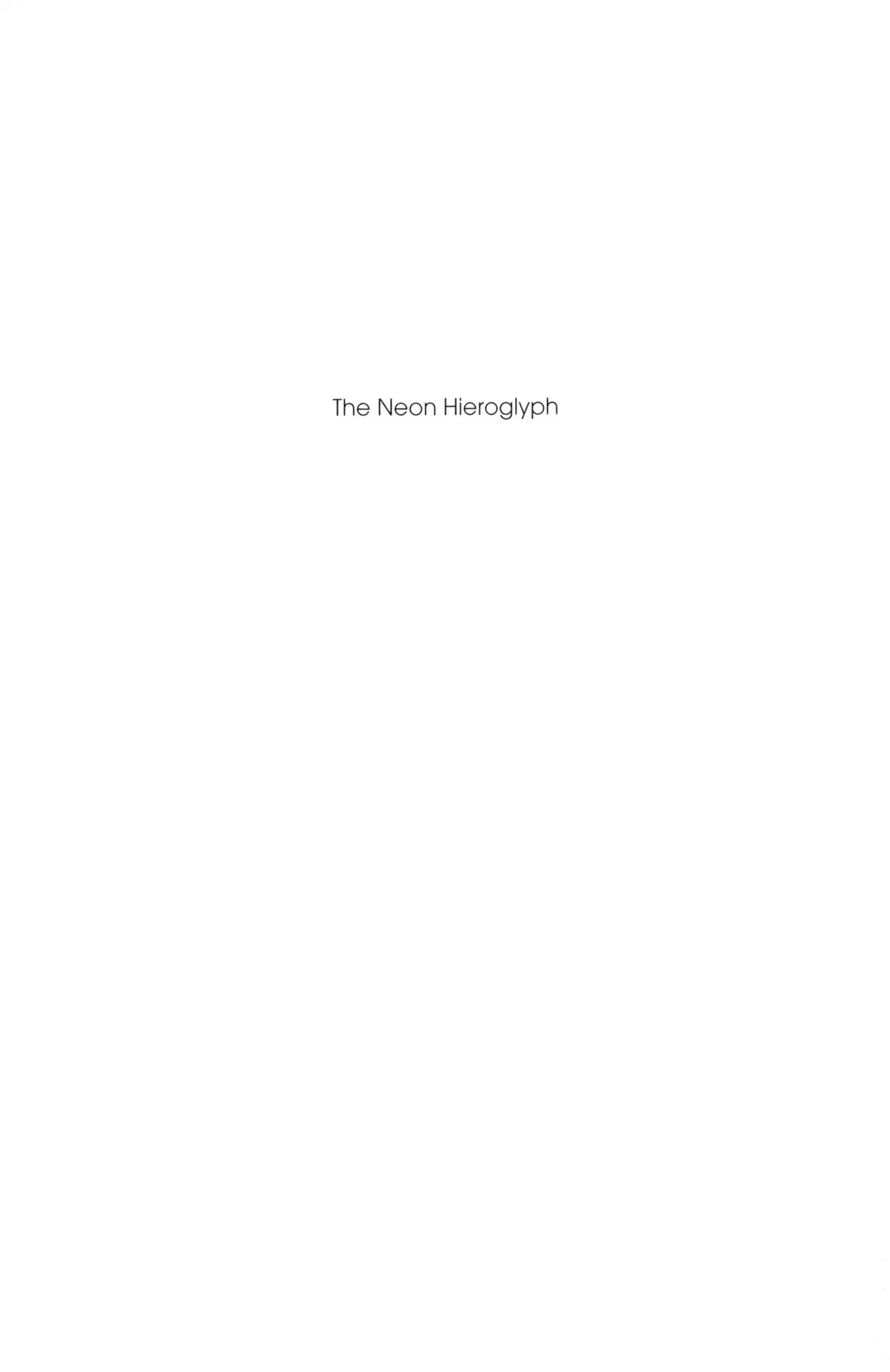

The Neon Hieroglyph

The Neon Hieroglyph
By Tai Shani
First published by Strange Attractor Press in 2022

ISBN: 9781913689490

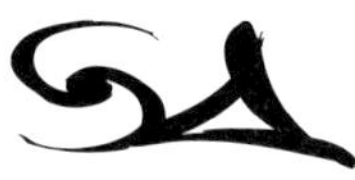

Distributed by The MIT Press, Cambridge, Massachusetts. And London, England.

Printed and bound in Estonia by Tallinna Raamatutrükikoda

Strange Attractor Press
BM SAP, London, WC1N 3XX UK
www.strangeattractor.co.uk

The Neon Hieroglyph

Tai Shani

Strange Attractor Press

Contents

"The Unbroken Cycle Of Our Interdependency"

Amy Hale

When Tai Shani calls me comrade, it feels warm and happy, like I have been injected with melted butter. Although the term has a rich political history of usage, some might even say baggage, for me it emphasizes a loving, relational quality, an acknowledgement that we are all in this together. It suggests the potential for unity, for care. Your comrade looks you square in the eye and takes your arm in partnership. Although *The Neon Hieroglyph* is, on the surface, a wildly decentered psychedelic ride of mythic histories through time and space, the deeper message, for me, is about our collective liberation and the web of connections uniting our shared fate; all beings through space, time and dimension, eternal comrades.

In contrast to the historical moment that sees us all bearing the persistent contusions of fear, confusion and lack of certainty, our circumstances dangerously marred by discourses of individual liberty taking precedence over the common good, I want to draw attention to the hopeful potentials seeded by *The Neon Hieroglyph*. In particular, the way it calls for us to see ourselves differently, as part of a much bigger, pulsating constellation of forces and energies. Perhaps now, more than ever, we need to embrace a condition characterized by the interdependence that has always been our often-unacknowledged reality, and, to paraphrase Donna Haraway, "wallow in multispecies muddles".

The Neon Hieroglyph exists in several states; text, performance, installation, and painting, expanding and contracting like a vital, autonomous universe, allowing the audience to encounter its key concepts and imagery from a variety of angles and dispersed settings. At its core, the project is about a mythic history of ergot, a fungus typically found on rye grain that causes hallucinations and visions when consumed, the alkaloids of which were eventually synthesized into LSD by the Swiss chemist Albert Hofmann in 1938. However, unlike ayahuasca or peyote, the consumption of ergot in its natural state is not typically linked to a contemporary, formalized ritual ingestion, and it happens by accident more than design, for example by eating bread which has been contaminated with ergot infected rye.

Within the context of women's health, ergot has been more conventionally described as an abortifacient and migraine treatment. Its unofficial effects, however, are linked to historical tales of underworld initiations, witches, astral travel, demons, dances of possession, and the communal folding of reality, all themes knotted together in Shani's work. The guiding text is arranged into nine visionary vignettes, each exploring an encounter with ergot. They move in a nonlinear manner from microcosmic to macrocosmic views, through the fictioning of historic moments, charting the expanses between spores and galaxies. Although *The Neon Hieroglyph* references specific histories and locales, the temporal narrative is effectively disjointed, simulating time travel through the psychedelic eyes of the narrator. Ergot is not just a tool or catalyst, it is an actor, an entity with its own story and memory.

The particular journey of *The Neon Hieroglyph* starts in the French village of Pont-Saint-Esprit, where an ergot outbreak blamed on cursed bread poisoned 250 people in August of 1951. Other tales include a colourful, hallucinatory version of the Eleusinian mysteries, as Kykeon, the barley wine ingested during the rites, is believed to have included ergot as a component, leading to visionary states. We will also meet ergot fueled manic dancers with bloody feet, communist witches, an orgasmic ergot spore moving through different hosts like a fungal Taliesin, and of course, dreaming androids.

The Neon Hieroglyph is, again, after Haraway, a work of 'speculative feminism', a feminist reworking of a psychedelic narrative, breaking the mold of the genre by divesting itself of linear notions of time, story or subject. It does not chronicle a singular change in state from one thing to another. It characterizes a pulsing meshwork of consciousness. Shani draws inspiration for this project from an influential 1937 British Science fiction classic, Olaf Stapledon's *Star Maker*. *Star Maker* is itself a beautifully psychedelic text, written during a time of incredible division and fear, featuring brilliant cosmic interconnected mind-melds, suggesting a new way of understanding the self in a web of relations.

> *"We", "Us", and "our" could be a cosmic community that connects time and space.*

Shani's feminist recasting of the psychedelic genre rejects the heroic journey of the rugged individualist, reinjecting themes of communality and of psychedelically envisioned conditions of welfare and care. The normative account of the counterculture psychedelic quest is most typically that of a man, a white man, using psychedelics, often or ideally facilitated by a cultural other, undergoing a deep, transformative experience. As Maggie Nelson has observed,[1] male drug narratives are heroic in character, with the male subjects escaping domesticity and socialization, rejecting responsibility and the collective in order to discover their authentic selves. After their enlightened transformation through the catalyst of the drug experience, they can rejoin the collective or reject it entirely, finding it corrupt. On the other hand, women's drug narratives are typically essentially degenerate, lacking the potential for a heroic arc. Women cannot abandon the domestic or the collective in any way that is not a moral failing. *The Neon Hieroglyph* is not, strictly speaking, a woman's drug narrative, although that particular genre is not irrelevant to the cultural positioning of this text. In many ways, this isn't a typical psychedelic narrative at all, and it is not a story about a single drug experience. Rather than abandoning the collective, the figures of *The Neon Hieroglyph* are swimming in it. As Shani explains:

> That sense of collectivity was the main thing I wanted to explore, and Ergot just seemed like a very interesting conduit for me to address how the more metaphysical questions, or the immaterial mysticism, or the fantastical dimensions of our lived experience or culture can be put to use in a more direct, social-materialist way.[2]

In recentering mutuality over the individual, the mythic, as opposed to the authored narrative, becomes the connective tissue of *The Neon Hieroglyph*. Myth and mythmaking has been an important element in Shani's corpus. She used the idiom of the mythic in *DC Productions*, a project which ran from 2014 to 2019, using Christine de Pizan's 1405 *Book of the City of Ladies* as a starting point, a text which itself is a story of a gathering of mythic women through place and time, disrupting linear history.

Myths are sacred stories of the people, beyond authorship, created by no one, and belonging to all. A story attains a status as mythic because it emerges from the anonymized collective. The central quality of myth that differentiates it from legend or history is that myths are big stories that tell us about central experiences of nature, culture, humanity. They are, by definition, stories that shape us; fictional yet deeply true. That which connotes the mythic often evokes the deep past, the past so far away in time that we cannot even apprehend its temporal locality. In *The Neon Hieroglyph*, however, Shani moves away from the temporal ideation of myth, instead focusing on the slippery nature between history and the big cultural stories that myth suggests. In *The Neon Hieroglyph*, myth can be located anywhere in time, inspiration may be drawn from the past or the future, and most certainly the present. Here, myths are not pulled from a golden age of the past, and let's face it, the past was never golden. Instead, Shani's mythic spaces can inspire from anywhere, emphasizing the inherent timelessness of myth as a category of story.

> *Below, above, the earth is a site for mythmaking and the collapse of myth into prosaic materials both natural and synthetic.*

Although myth is popularly understood as having been generated in an ahistorical past, commentators such as Barthes and Breton observe that the power of myth lies in the greatness and relevance of the story, not its origin in imagined time. Thus, *The Neon Hieroglyph* as a liberatory exercise exists in a tension: Stories from the past are powerful, and there are many forgotten or marginalized stories which need to be told. Yet we also need to be liberated from the cultural paradigms of the past that oppress us, by creating spaces for new myths and models to emerge. In weaving these stories of ergot and women together, Shani offers us the possibility of creating new myths and looking at other forgotten stories through different lenses.

But what does it mean to create new myths? In his 1942 'Prolegomena to a Third Surrealist Manifesto (or Not)', André Breton questions the central role of myth in society and asks how we can free ourselves of the confines of potent narratives that no longer suit us: "What should one think of the postulate that 'there is no society without a social myth'? In what measure can we choose or adopt, and impose, a myth fostering the society that we judge to be desirable?" How can we even know what that society looks like when we are so imaginatively steeped in models that we don't want to reproduce?

Although Shani is not responding to Mark Fisher's *Capitalist Realism* in any formal way, *The Neon Hieroglyph* takes as part of its premise the notion that our world is so saturated by capitalism and the political discourses and structures that sit in opposition to it, that we require other modes of being to escape this stranglehold on our psyches and our resistance. Shani proposes that when we enter psychedelic spaces we can call into being structures and relationships that are unnamed and untouched by an all pervasive capitalist reality. Again, turning to Fisher, his unfinished *Acid Communism* (in part derived from research by Jeremy Gilbert), only hints at a solution that Shani articulates within a framework distinguished by feminist aesthetics and unboundedness. While Fisher seems somewhat wistful for the unfulfilled potential of the psychedelic counterculture, Shani locates the promise of psychedelic experience in neither past nor future, but suggests its existence may be productively timeless, sustained in imaginative potential.

> *When AIs dream, they dream in uninhibited psychedelics.*

The Neon Hieroglyph introduces us to figures and moments that become liberatory because of how we are encouraged to view them, and to view with them. We are connected by ways of seeing. Shani hints toward a ubiquitous psychedelic experience that we share with artificial intelligence, spores, and priestesses, seen in the squiggles and luminous abstractions of cave paintings, phosphenes, drug-induced journeys, and dreams. Thus, the images, and imagined experiences, of both organic and seemingly inorganic objects and materials are brought into novel proximities, while fragments of the past and the future collapse into each other.

> *Here too, even more determinedly, we felt we completed some fractal design, coded into the digital's hallucinogenic natural, and nature's analogue psychedelic.*

In each fragment we are brought back to shared visual experience, shared patterns, all of us born from the hearts of stars. Life transforms to death and back again, joy and repulsion are two sides of the same coin.

> *You are terrifying there, how beautiful you are, we all are, the baby's toes and the poor pea-hen, the spoon, the moonlight, and the flax, the spittle and the dust. In this flow, we are cusp-dwellers, constituted of stardust, only just holding back the panic with all this magnificent beauty and horror around us and in us too.*

The stories are undergirded by the power of those working in ecstasy for the shared good of all, the witches, the priestesses, the dancers, the orgasmic spores. The witch is the ultimate psychedelic figure in *The Neon Hieroglyph*, a symbol of resistance, confronting oppression and hierarchies with the ability to shift between planes and forms. Again, Shani:

> The witch is the human embodiment of chaotic wickedness and dark powers, and powerful she is but she is also a wrecker of civilisation and morality.[3]

In recent years the witch has gained new social standing as an outlaw figure, for whom magic and outsider status itself provide agency in a world where we often feel powerless. Images of the wise witch of the village, or of cunning folk inspire contemporary individualistic responses to late capitalism and the sense of relentless, perpetual disempowerment felt by so many. Yet Shani's witch as a figure of justice has a strong cultural pedigree that aligns magic with the ethics of communal welfare. In *The Neon Hieroglyph* the witch may act alone, but working for the collective she is a figure of redistribution, of levelling, of righteous power. Shani's witch, inspired by Italian folklore, is both a figure of liberation but also of bounty, with its own slightly different ethical trajectory. We see here the traces of La Befana, the Italian witch who delivers gifts and candy to children on Epiphany. We also see the radical coven of witches suggested by folklorist Charles Leland's 1899 *Aradia, or the Gospel of the Witches*, the seminal text also based on Italian accounts which inspired both the theology and the liturgy of modern Wicca.

The witches of *Aradia* are explicitly a coven of resistance acting against an oppressive class who has enslaved them. The work of witchcraft in this text is to bind and poison the ruling class. These witches have freed themselves from slavery, and as a sign of that freedom are naked when they meet. It is their job to help emancipate others.

> *We make circles of salt, we fly to the sleepy Calabrian towns to steal from the rich, we kiss with venomous serpents, we spell for revolution, we invoke the angels that course wildly in the elements.*

Above all, *The Neon Hieroglyph* isn't about evoking ideas of a past or future that will bring about our liberation, it is about recognizing the enduring entanglement of all; organic and inorganic, all beings freed from the illusory burden of believing that we are going it alone. We have inherited a narrative that reifies the concept of a discrete, bounded individualism that suggests that we are socially and biologically predisposed to a singular, unique mode of perception that is ours alone. But what would it mean for us to anticipate a shared vision, literally and psychedelically? Might that bring us to an understanding and a truer experience of our deep interconnection? In isolation and in darkness, can we rub our eyes and connect through time to those who recorded their own shining visions on the walls of caves?

> *The organic eye discloses autogenetic symbols on the backdrop of a midnight of light. Phosphenes, grids, filigree, spots, radiations, vitreous mosaics, prismatic halos, the movement of white blood cells in capillaries in front of the retina, floating coagulations of vitreous jelly within the eye. Once painted, become: a limonite zigzag, a hematite cluster of dots, a calcite reticulation, a charcoal halo.*

In "Notes Towards a Feminist Futurist Manifesto" Sarah Kember asks if it's time to be done with the future, given how limited, often uninspiring, or downright terrifying most contemporary visions of the future are. Kember suggests that a feminist futurism rejects linear histories with their thinly veiled ideologies of "progress":

> Feminist genealogies, in addition to genealogies of feminism, rather than deploying history against the future, engage it through an investment that is necessarily imaginative, even speculative, in the possibility of political change.[4]

This is the crux of the liberatory and feminist heart of *The Neon Hieroglyph*, resisting form, space, the impositions of historical authority. Although hope itself suggests a future state that I do not want to project into the meaning of the text, *The Neon Hieroglyph* makes me feel hopeful. I see it as about the potential in emergence, in rearranging, in unfolding, in becoming — an expression of concrescence. It is an invitation to remember where we have been; together in Eleusis, as spores, as tiny gods, as ghosts, and to remember all that we will be, linked together, enmeshed, eternally collaborating.

> *A prose-like network of cellular activity and phenomena, subtle mannerisms that provoke so much tenderness and eternal devotion, from one lost coordinate on the temporal plane to another.*

Notes

1. Maggie Nelson, *On Freedom: Four Songs of Care and Constraint*. Minneapolis: Graywolf Press, 2021.
2. Serpentine Gallery. "In Conversation: Tai Shani, Untitled Hieroglyphs" (https://www.serpentinegalleries.org/art-and-ideas/in-conversation-tai-shani-untitled-hieroglyphs/)
3. Email from Tai Shani to author, 28 January 2021.
4. Sarah Kember, "Notes Toward a Feminist Future Manifesto" in *ADA: A Journal of Gender, New Media and Technology* #1 2012 (https://adanewmedia.org/2012/11/issue1-kember/)

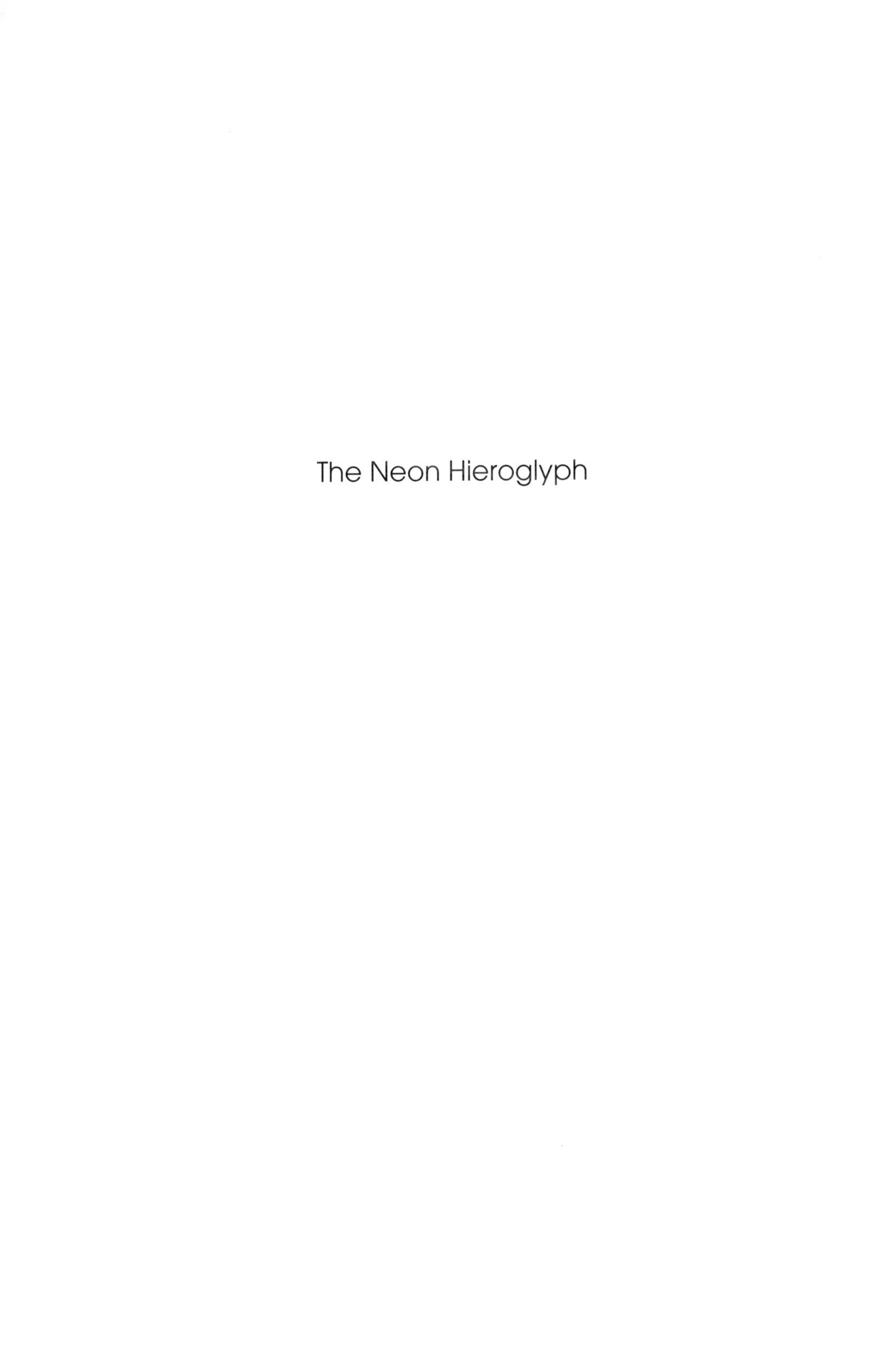

The Neon Hieroglyph

1

The sun is a ghost that haunts the night.

Pont-St-Esprit, 1951.

Clouds cross and catastrophise the sky, travel across catastrophes and love.

It was the hottest day of the year. The sky boiled, we coughed in gasps of scalding air, cauterising the wounds of our tongues. The air was completely still, everything outside was frozen in the choke of heat. The windows looked like photographs stuck on the walls of a crypt-like furnace.

We had eaten the poisonous bread, milled from contaminated rye.

"Do you too feel manic when you swell and are about to burst?" We ask the dragon, tiger, paisley, whey clouds.

Although we are completely ordinary, we are strange creatures too.

At the close of day, I look back at you from the coiling cold waters of a tidal river.

I is you, and you is whoever you choose.

Through a thick custard vape cloud and a constellation of suspended pollen, neck-deep in the layers and layers of nuclear family, pink and yellow tigers slither up from the dark waters onto the bank of the river.

The sky bursting full, whipped grey, an uneven strip of opal suspended carefully over you, an incandescent radiant tapestry, the polymorph, the dreaming androids, and seraphim above you. You lying loose on a towel, reading a book about chaos and fascist politics, "why now?" It was never not *why*, or *how*, on the yellowing grass that surged groaning, and then purringly withdrew. In the fresh water, I try to pull thousands of strands of silken hair that I can't grasp growing out of my mouth in a suburban park at the end of summer.

We had eaten the bread. The village children had eaten the bread. The thistle, the chamomile, the nettle, the rosehip, the primrose, the hellebore, the immense blackberry bush. The children, beads of pearlescent water falling from them, their wet hair slicked down like the duck's tail, pick off the fruit with their berry-stained fingers and learn the very little they will ever know about the natural world.

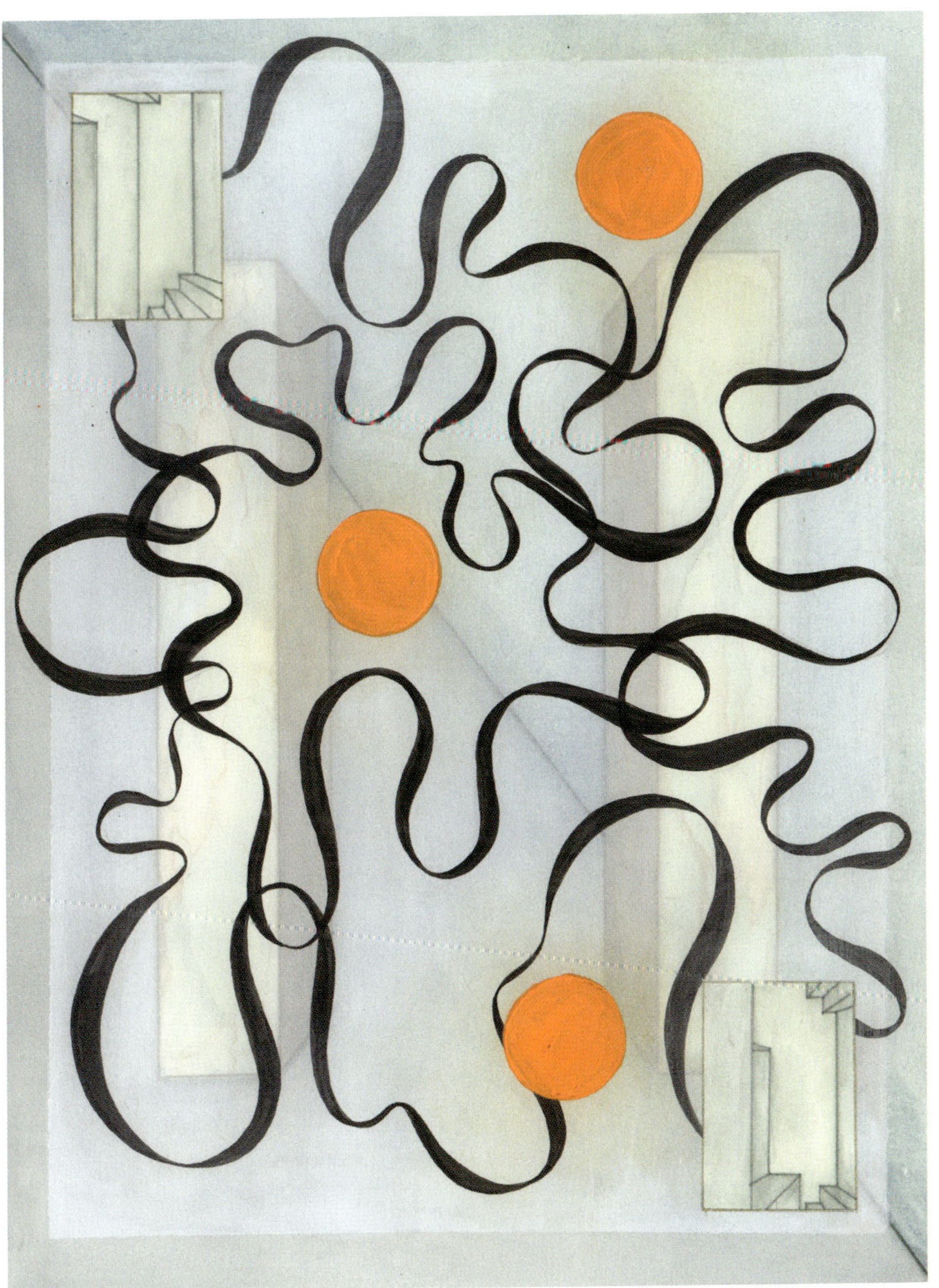

2

"Please do not be afraid of the dead, it is only the living that can and will certainly hurt us," they said, before opening the heavy door of the crypt, CAVE ENTRANCE the entrance into the lightless, telestic chamber, which could possibly be endless in its conclusive quiet and inexhaustible darkness.

To fear the supernatural is to make theatre out of our fear of our capacity for violence — violence of indifference to violence of inexhaustible cruelty; a fear of fascism, and the spookiest of all fears, the fear of our powerlessness.

In the Inner Eye is a blueprint of the common visual language of psychotropics, trances, channeling, and artificial intelligence, when pushed to its limits — a dreamstate. When AIs dream, they dream in uninhibited psychedelics.

We travel through three lightless spaces, which in their darkness are interchangeable.

A crypt with photographs of the world on its walls, to not forget, in the house for the forgotten dead, a home for our undead, a bed for our vampire's plasmatic recoveries. Our zombies emerge ravenous for your un-undead flesh. Our melancholic phantoms, terminally fused to passages of their lived lives, passages of unspeakable trauma, unspeakable joy.

No peace, no respite for the spirit separated, as that of our phantom's body left to a submission to atomic extinction, it decomposes inside the crypt before our disembodied sight, as our time moves forward, forward, forward relentlessly. The dead — we are so alike.

In the cell, across the eyes, a blind screen of abstract luminous hallucinations appears after extended periods of sensory deprivation. They call it "Prisoner's Cinema". In the ethical abomination that is the carceral state, a prisoner who is deprived of all contact in solitary confinement physically attacks the brutal pig of a warden to experience some form of touch.

Deprived of visual stimulation, hallucinated vivid lights sometimes transition from abstraction to figuration and characters are formed. On occasion, they can even play out narratives such as this.

In the cave, past the sweeping fadeout of light, before world was painted: the bison, the hunt, and the hands. Painted in limonite, hematite, calcite, and charcoal, a record of cryptic optic messages traced from the slippery retinal wall onto the limestone wall of the cave.

The organic eye discloses autogenetic symbols on the backdrop of a midnight of light. Phosphenes, grids, filigree, spots, radiations, vitreous mosaics, prismatic halos, the movement of white blood cells in capillaries in front of the retina, floating coagulations of vitreous jelly within the eye. Once painted, become: a limonite zigzag, a hematite cluster of dots, a calcite reticulation, a charcoal halo.

We wept psychic tears in the crypt, under the disclosing glass eye of the microscope. Collected psychic tears are aerial maps, oils, antibodies and enzymes suspended in salt water. There are crystal bricks with which to build a glassy mausoleum, to build the temple where we descended on the solstice, to build the most powerful city in the world, now the ruins in an archaeological site that we wept from myth into the real.

A fourth unidentified, lightless place.

Disassociated, terrible reality did not feel real at all. All the rose emojis at the end of each message were making us cry. The impermanence became marked phenotypically across our faces, our eyes continuously pooled, our awed, gaping mouths fell almost silent, apart from a creepy note of parasitic panic humming subtly beneath death tolls and other ambient noise.

It was a war, it always had been.

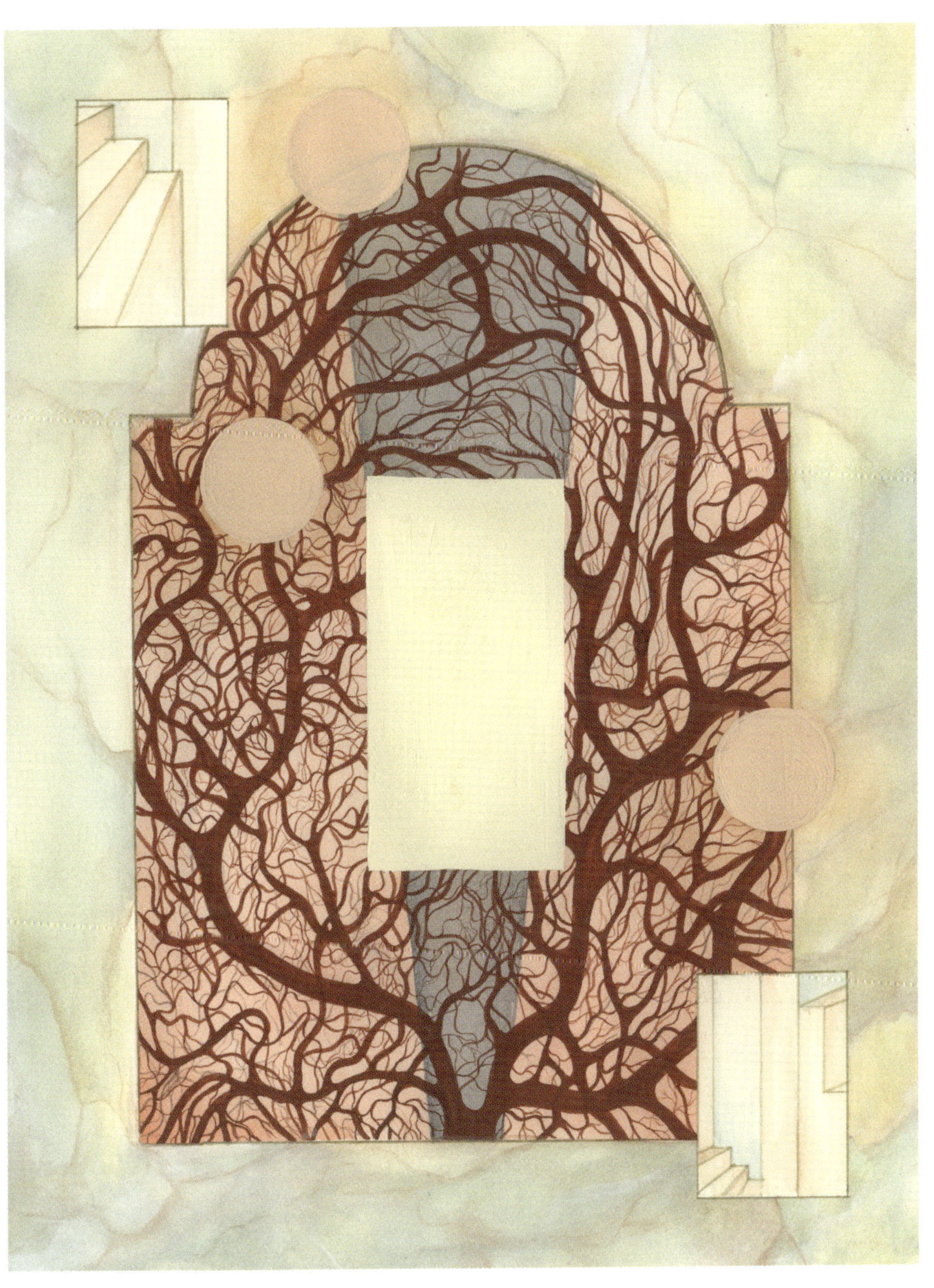

3

House, Table, Dog, Fire.

We are green, green atoms. Green atoms become green electrons, then green protons and neutrons, which become green quarks.

We are phytoplankton, greenly photosynthesize into photosensitive green life givers. We would be eternally green communists, eternally horizontal, eternally porous, eternally communing to collaboratively compose the epic unsung anthem of the unbroken cycle of our interdependency. A fragile ecology in the powerful movements of astral dust.

We wait for an eternity under a green spiritual spotlight in the metaphysical proscenium arch — our eyes closed, dispersing the density of the neon hieroglyphs, skittering towards the contrast of the dim periphery of the eye — to become visible again.

Here too, even more determinedly, we felt we completed some fractal design, coded into the digital's hallucinogenic natural, and nature's analogue psychedelic.

The sexual and asexual reproduction of fungus that grows parasitically on common grains, which contain alkaloids from which LSD can be derived.

It was time, our fruiting bodies, abundant and excessive, our pollinated ovaries, our multiple spores brimming. We were club-headed, erect, and swelling. We survived the winter on sterile rye in the face of the deficient copper in the soil, and germinated, reproducing both asexually and sexually, bound together by the sticky sap, to make pathogenetic neon hieroglyphic, code-writer fungus.

In the sticky sap, I came sexually and asexually, and when I came I was a brain-eating alien. I was a snapped stalactite, I was your quivering shadow, I was a roundworm larvae carried by a sick pig in an industrial farm, I was shimmer, I was idle, I was a distant bark.

When I came, I cried in karyogamic bliss to all the quarks that realised my pleasure, my unbreachable distance from my name, from my culture, from my history.

June, 2020.

"You will die," we whisper in your ear, sitting on your chest.

We rip open your pink playdough face for an anthropomantic divination of an encrypted future in your spilling carmine wound, which was once your necropolitical face on a thousand police cars set ablaze, in the streets of our beloved paradisiac Hell House.

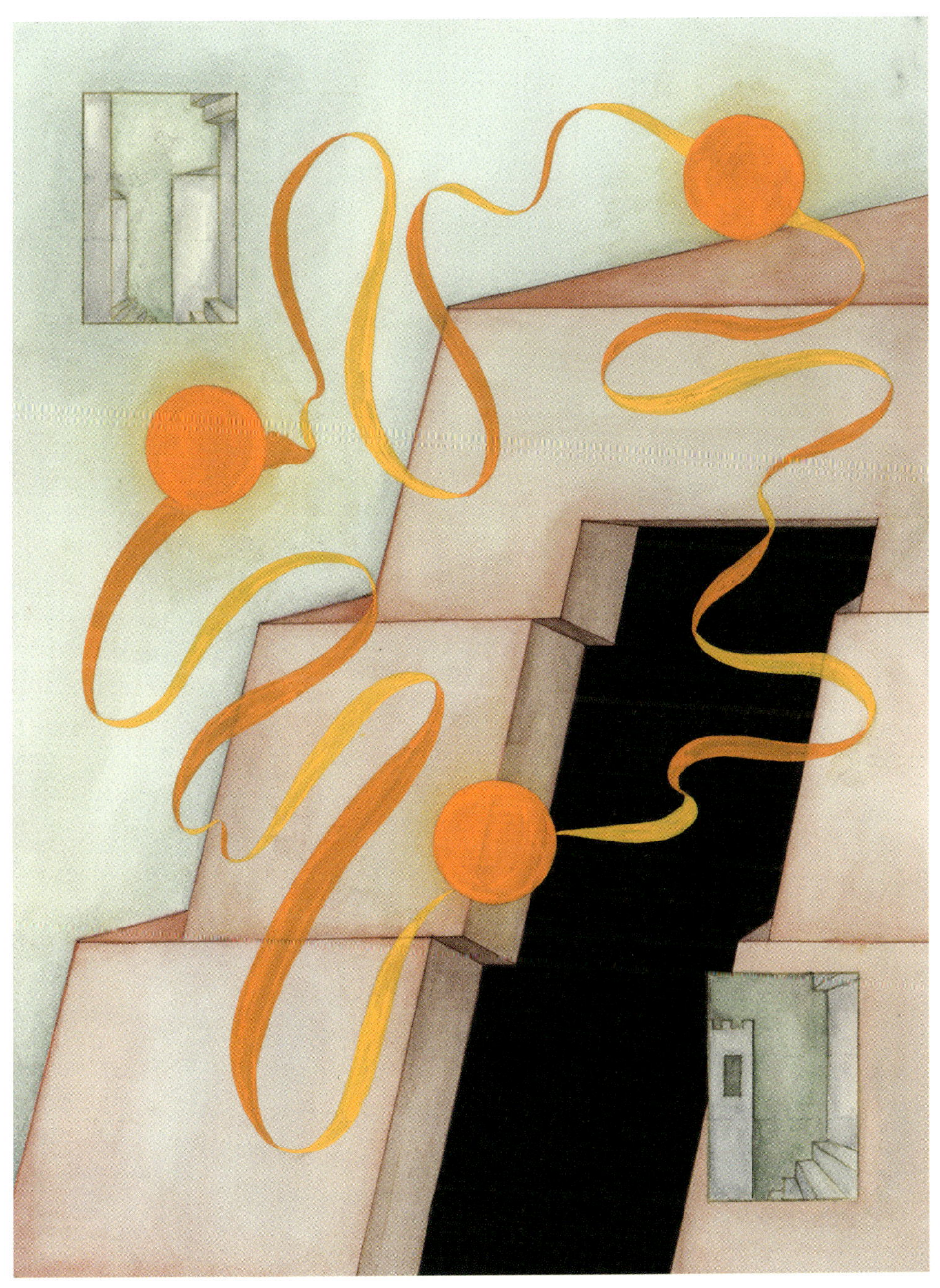

4

The Dancing Plagues and other afflictions.

"We", "Us", and "our" could be a cosmic community that connects time and space.

When we stop, and stand still, our insides drop, the muscles in our thighs spasm repeatedly.

Tiny shudders, like muscles under silken stallion coats, green, blue, purple, twitch, and flies levitate softly, into floating clouds of somnambulists, jewelled in the caught light, a thousand lenses in five eyes.

Our feet settle into a red raw pain. Blood and sweat make a sticky sap that soaks into the dead leather of our shoes and stings our tenderized flesh.

When we stop, the world is still moving, our bodies are painful, the world is unbearable, cannot contain us, is about to spit us out into a yawning mouth of inconsolable sadness to be swallowed and dissolved by spleen's acid into useless small chunks that sometimes appear floating in vomit.

The expanding pattern of grass and small pebbles and sky and earth, tendrils, hairs weaving into a textured surface perpetually, almost a face, almost a shoe, almost rain, almost objects, almost subjects, subjects that just deserve so much better than this cradle to grave brutality, what can I say.

When we dance, the pain of our muscles and joints, the thirst in our mouths and throats vanishes in the throb of a blurry sensation subsumed in the rhythm of the movement. We are lifted and stirred by a motion that animates all.

Within that motion, we touch and are touched by a harmony in which nothing is out of step, nothing can cause pain. Pain itself is outside of the rhythm, reliant on a strict measure that does not exist here, nor does the measure of work, the state, of the evil forces that govern our lives. And here we lived a life in the fundamental love that they cannot contaminate, we lived a thousand real lives, we protected and were all worthy of protection.

You are terrifying there, how beautiful you are, we all are, the baby's toes and the poor pea-hen, the spoon, the moonlight, and the flax, the spittle and the dust. In this flow, we are cusp-dwellers, constituted of stardust, only just holding back the panic with all this magnificent beauty and horror around us and in us too.

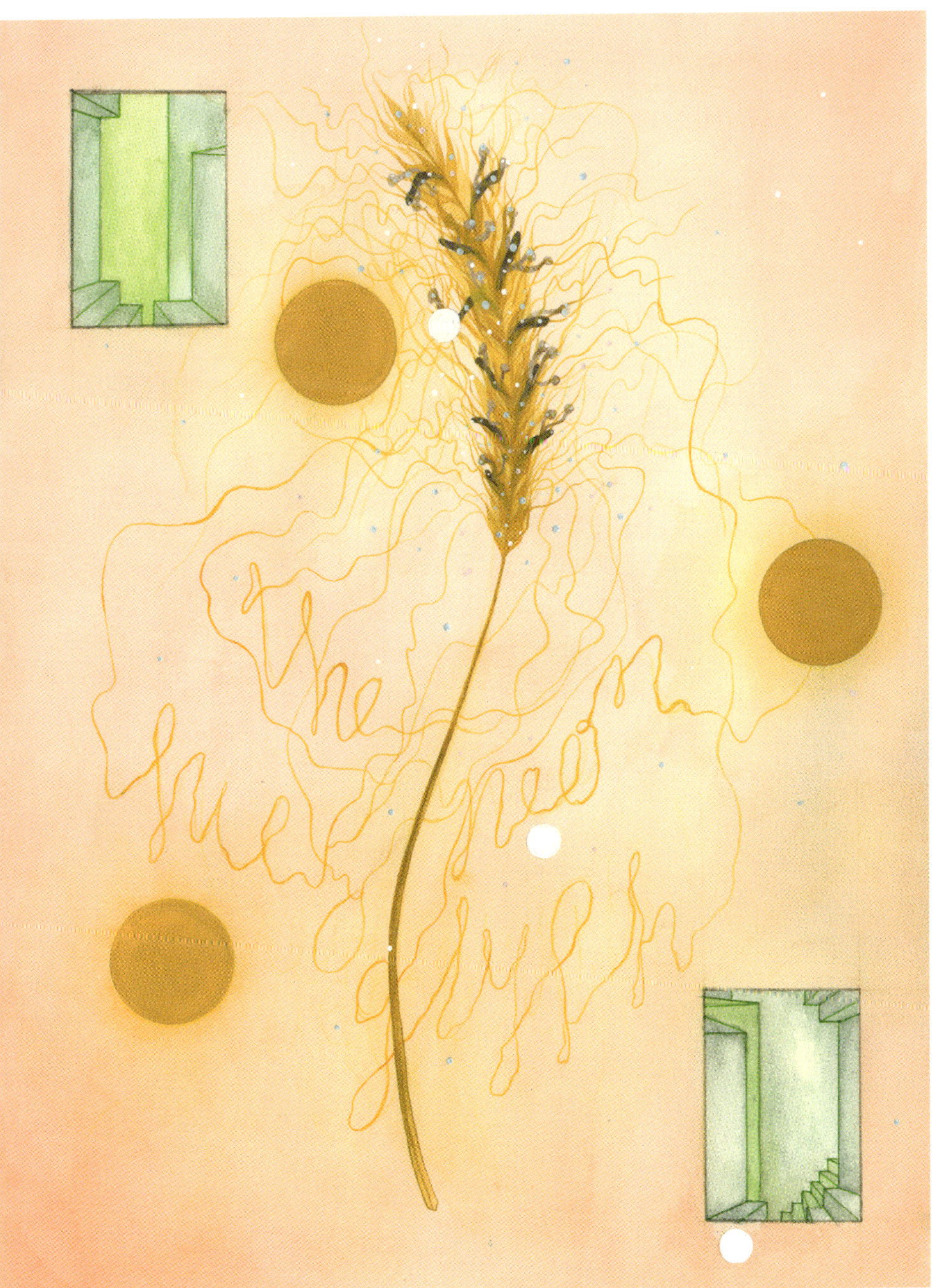
the
hue neon
glyph

5

Persephone's descent to into the dark of the underworld reaches a cusp, where it inverts and transforms into an ascent from the underworld into the light.

It is time to say goodbye. Your funeral will be your faery name spelt in a murmuration pattern at dusk. They promised us.

Down, Rharian field, ellipses, carnivores, swanskin, and poplin. Consumed spoiled grain fatally atrophies, in muted purple, the useful limbs, and tessellates fractals that bridge into worlds unknown where our grasp on a telepathic, interdependent language is sensual.

Soundwaves can only travel as long as their molecular collaborators will carry them, where they will end up in a museum of unrecoverable vibrations.

Down, skin, pelt, vellum, alert tangled roots, subcutaneous flesh, subterranean blind life, my bodily remains, your bodily remains, and all the bodily remains that ever were, and ever will be.

Down, coal and gold in the rocks, a coughed ash cloud. Gold production in the Universe is present in the dust from which this Solar System formed.

Gold, yellow, but will not go clear like butter does in the heat. Into the gold extracted with cyanide.

Bitter almonds, cassava, Zyklon B, cherry stone, apple seed, in the smoke of combusting plastics, in the production of paper and textiles, in the stabilising of the photographic image on paper.

Gold ring of Saturn rubbed against a stye on a puffy red eyelid. Eyelash fans shut. Venus flytrap, beneath neon hieroglyph and solar pulse, yellow, golden glow.

Gold heirloom, white gold cocktail watch for scrap metal, melted white gold, will not go clear like snow in first light. Forever night white gold.

Our mouths open, my tongue deep in your mouth against a gold filling of a dead, unnerved, tooth. In this erotic kiss we are resurrected, my tongue pressed against your unresurrectable biology. Baby Osiris.

Down, into the source of the well, we all drink from, it binds to iron in our blood. Liquid biopowerful poisons travel up through the compacted earth, corroding and seeping into the system of pipes, and flush through the mouths and nipples of marble gods and heroes, flowing directly into their mouths. They drink.

Baby Osiris in the underworld asks about those technocratic desires. Ours are stone age desires, so hot, molten lava, from the molten core of the world spitting out magma into the cosmic spray of the galaxy.

We are sucked into the core, bloodless, past the gates and into the flaming heat of haematic hellmouth, the deathless eternal endurance of the burning of the abyssal fire.

Survived and up, up, transformed, towards the light, through the other side, through gold again and platinum, through the mesospheric mantle, through the waning primordial heat and decaying radioactivity of uranium. Up, into the softening, liquidising rocks of the asthenosphere, past the diamond mines, travelling up through the compacted earth.

Counteragents in the system of sarcoline pipes, our lips and tongues will push through the mouths and nipples of marble gods and heroes to suck the poison out of rubious fleshmouths, as from fatal snakebites.

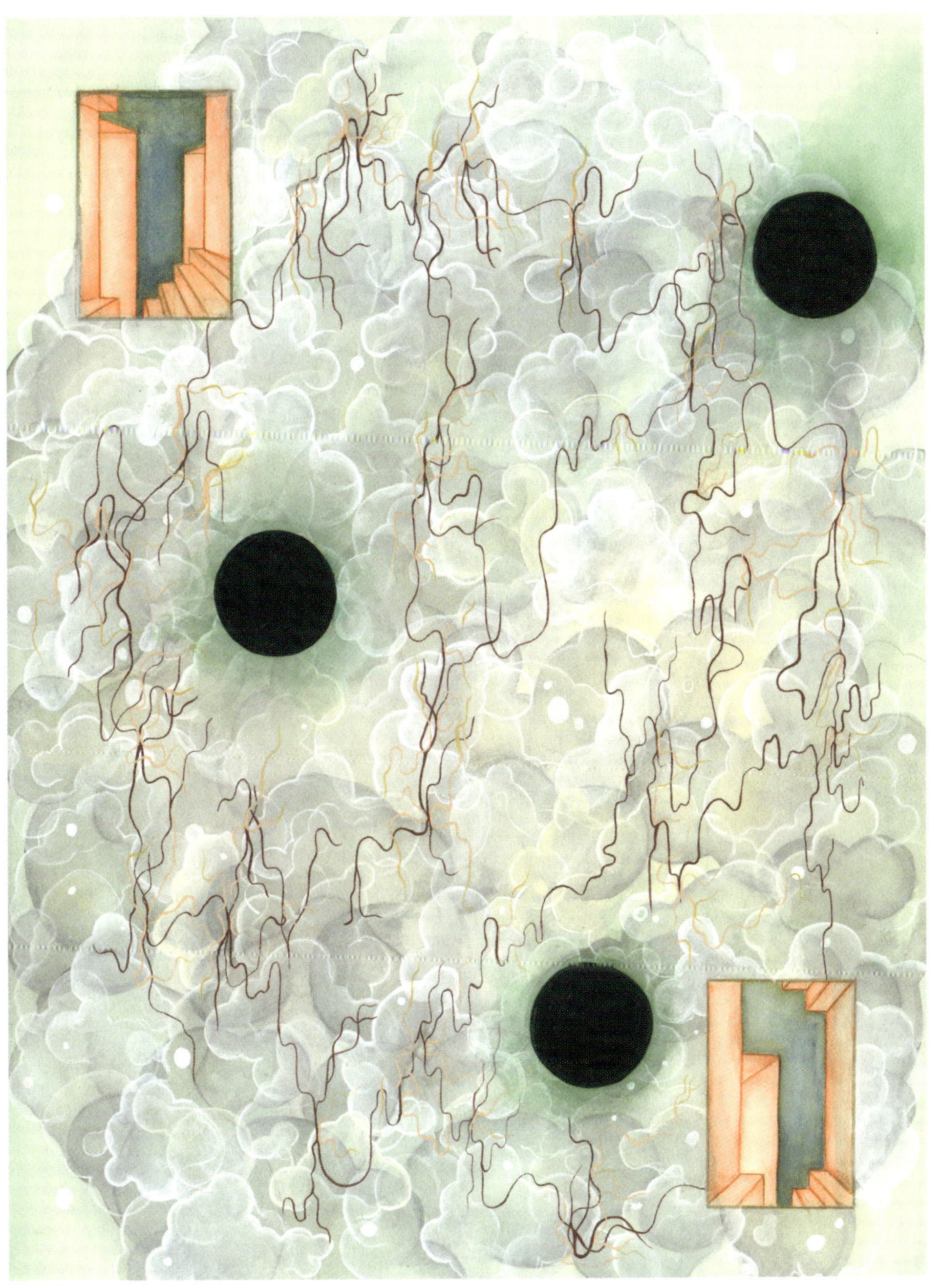

6

Alicudi, Aeolian Islands, 1862.

This bread is a placebo, the bread is a spaceship.

Gothic sea-sides, breached nebula, fabric rustle, birdsong, bark, air, and breath echoes into a psychogenic, fractal decomposition. Our fractal love, our fractal dread: we see you, we make and are made by you.

We will still be here in the disintegration of us, which leaves an unfolding of luminous, ibis-feathered, haloed trails around our movements. We say tetragrammatic words of the mystics and triptych images of the patronised artists, trinities holy and unholy, from the borderlands of Hell House, with its garden envenomed by the overgrown oleander bushes. You, me and us. We will all find decay in the perished remains of their corrupt architecture.

In the electronic rush of a constant beat we hear a constant horizon. We see in the constant horizon a mausoleum for the psychedelic witches. We paint our bodies with the Oleander oil, like Persephone painted all the flowers of the world. We make circles of salt, we fly to the sleepy Calabrian towns to steal from the rich, we kiss with venomous serpents, we spell for revolution, we invoke the angels that course wildly in the elements.

159 years later.

We summon the tiny animistic gods that imbue wood with its woodness, the tiny gods that render sulphur sulphuric, the tiny gods of wood transformed into tiny gods of paper, the tiny gods of glue, the tiny gods of sand melted to become tiny gods of glass that has been crushed, and they now mingle with tiny red gods of phosphorus, to make a surface for that match to strike and ignite. They call upon the many tiny furious gods of the fire, and we will throw that match and watch the tiny gods furiously burn their whole lifetaking, infernal world down, and we will see each other's smiles in the light of that fire.

This bread is real, it kills heroes. This bread is a starmaker of collected stardust.

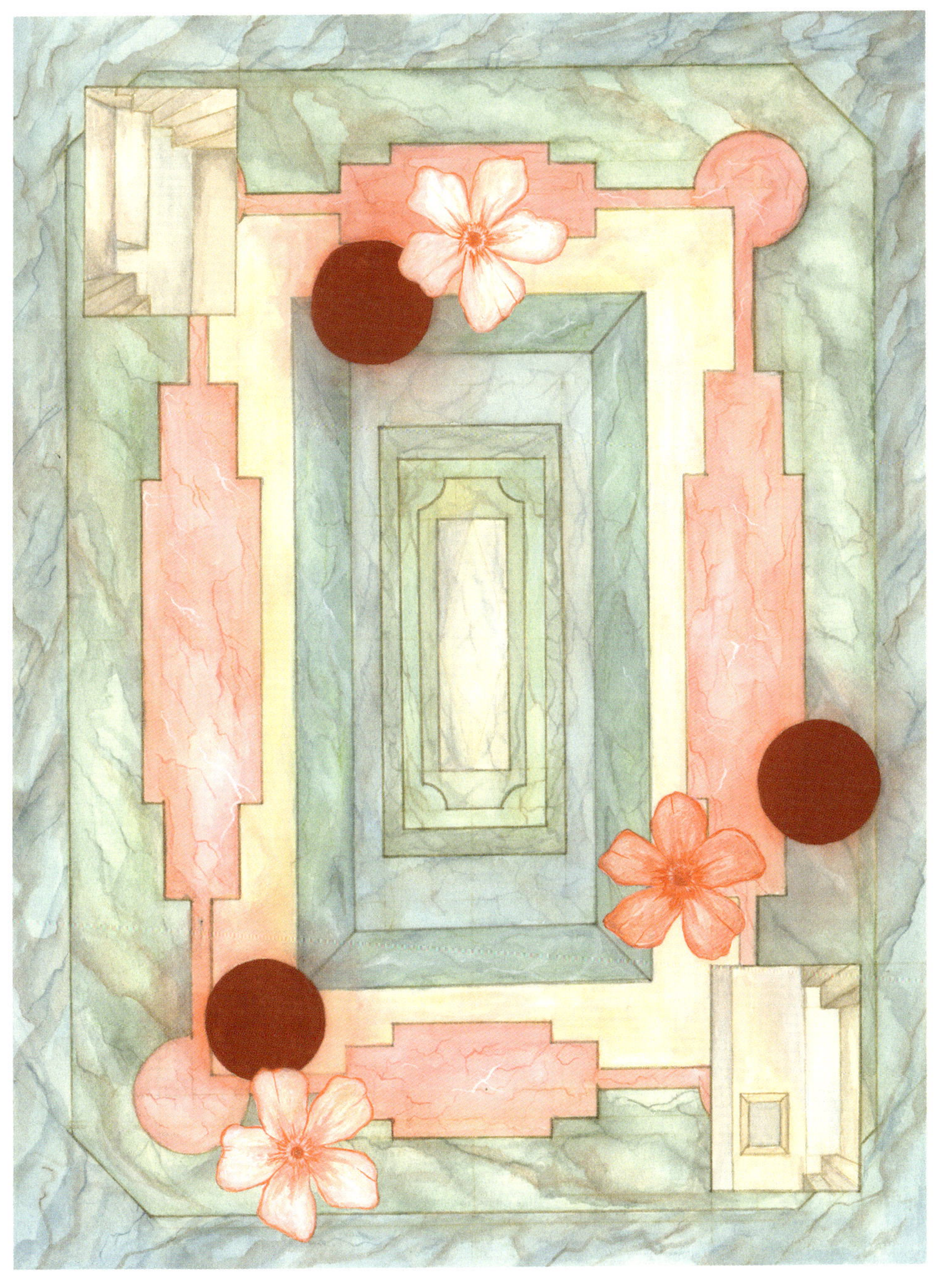

7

A drone aerial vista.

This is the birth of cinema.

"This is the death of cinema," scratched into the holographic surface of a DVD, of *It Happened Tomorrow*.

Yes, it was the day the world went Day-Glo.

We exchanged spectacularized ocular fluids continuously, mouth to mouth, watertight, the screen and us, hewing grooves for the fluids to douse and drain, to and from each other.

Oh, how we touched.

Digital eye, binary code left us trapped, undone and disjointed, threw us into the contested borders between our world and theirs, unable to enter either.

We live and fly like the sirens, in searching sadness, wanting a true retributive justice.

In horrors and thrillers, in the forest they ran for their lives, they drove away never looking back from the scene of the crime. Their laughter or their terrified screams spilled out from their mouths, beat against the rocky hill, through the crown-shy trees, close to the grooming tiger in the sugarcane and the magnetic forcefield of Hanuman's sacred temple.

Them, them, eyes clear, high out of their minds, high, high, high, up to where the edelweiss grows purer and wilder, climbing up to paradise.

Euphoric and erratic, a crying Pierrot postcard in the jeep, splicing western iconography into this deep, transformative night – how can I not be thankful for this? We lived a thousand lives, close to the flame, those days and nights.

My eyes, you broke my heart.

A liberated organ, an eye thrown up into the thinness and clarity of the atmosphere, haunting a new landscape built from eruptive tectonic shifts of land and relics of obsolete technologies.

A thousand drones flew overhead, capturing the script of topographies natural and designed on the ground, also, I thought, in sky. We levitated, became ghosts. We haunted the earth, we were purgatorial agents; and we also ascended, floating above our world, between worlds, suspended in passage from one realm to another.

It was silent, it was black and white, it was viral, it was aerial. They travelled above, captured a teleported view. The eyes in the sky tore open a modest dimension in which I could momentarily deep-dream that I was able to be there again, and this time it would not be the same.

Below every surface a miracle, every cell contingent on a series of miracles.

When you were a small child, you would run to me and throw your arms around me sweetly and say, "full of love!", before, like most of us, you were completely destroyed by terrible and unfair circumstances beyond your control, beyond anyone's control. Little learner's arms around me, your open, antidote face pushed into my stomach.

Full of love, yes I felt it too, the antidote as viral as the disease.

Trust me. Tonight we will suppress the dull workings of a pessimistic and worried mind. We will listen till the patterns coalesce into algorithmic, translucent tapestries, all animate and inanimate breathe in unison, and the polymorph, the dreaming androids and seraphim appear in flames.

Then we will fly.

Now we are as light as a newborn, we will fly like phantasma, fly like the sirens in searching sadness, and find a true retributive justice. We will fly like the bewitched, above the highway, the curling road, the dirt road that glows dazzlingly in the summer months with a thousand fireflies, the unmapped, foreboding path that will bring us to the house where we once all had to live, were eternally stained.

And we will haunt and be haunted by that moment of true delight, we will be overwhelmed till no part of me can breathe from the sincerity of this love that ran so freely through you.

My eyes, you broke my heart.

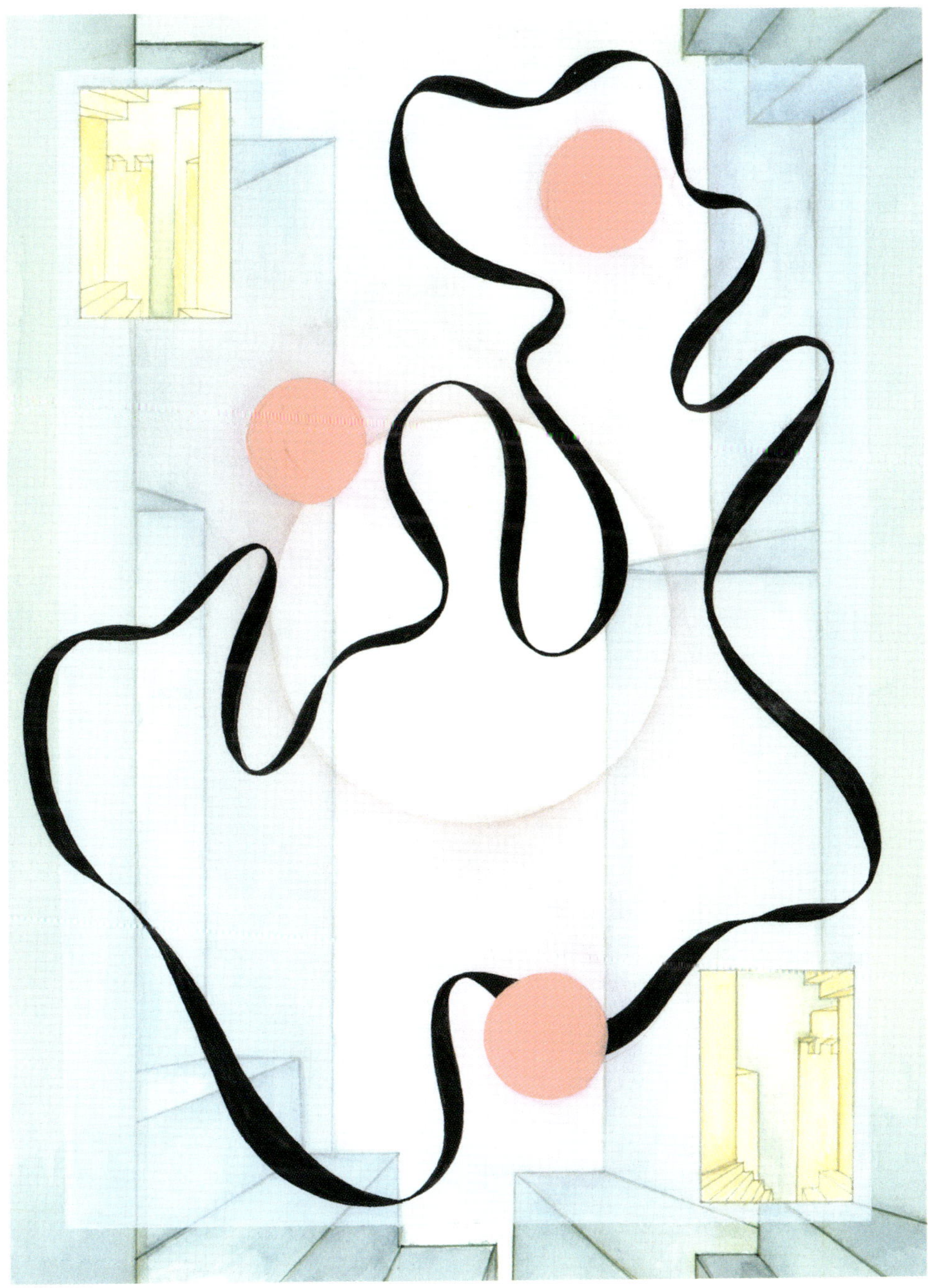

8

Happy birthday to the celestial bodies above, scribbled metaphysical toilet graffiti inside.

Below, above, the earth is a site for mythmaking and the collapse of myth into prosaic materials both natural and synthetic.

From our world, we hold a mirror to the sun, tilt it back and forwards and send an important message in simple code. Are you receiving?

All we hear is midnight birdsong on the longest night of the year.

Sounds like the end of the world when birds sing in the deep darkness.

For little photosensitive robins in the city, the end of day never comes. They sing at night because of the sprawling noise. In the dark and quiet night, their song might be heard. To sing, they expend vast amounts of energy, almost die, but it must be heard. They sing to let each other know they are here, they are alive, and that is all.

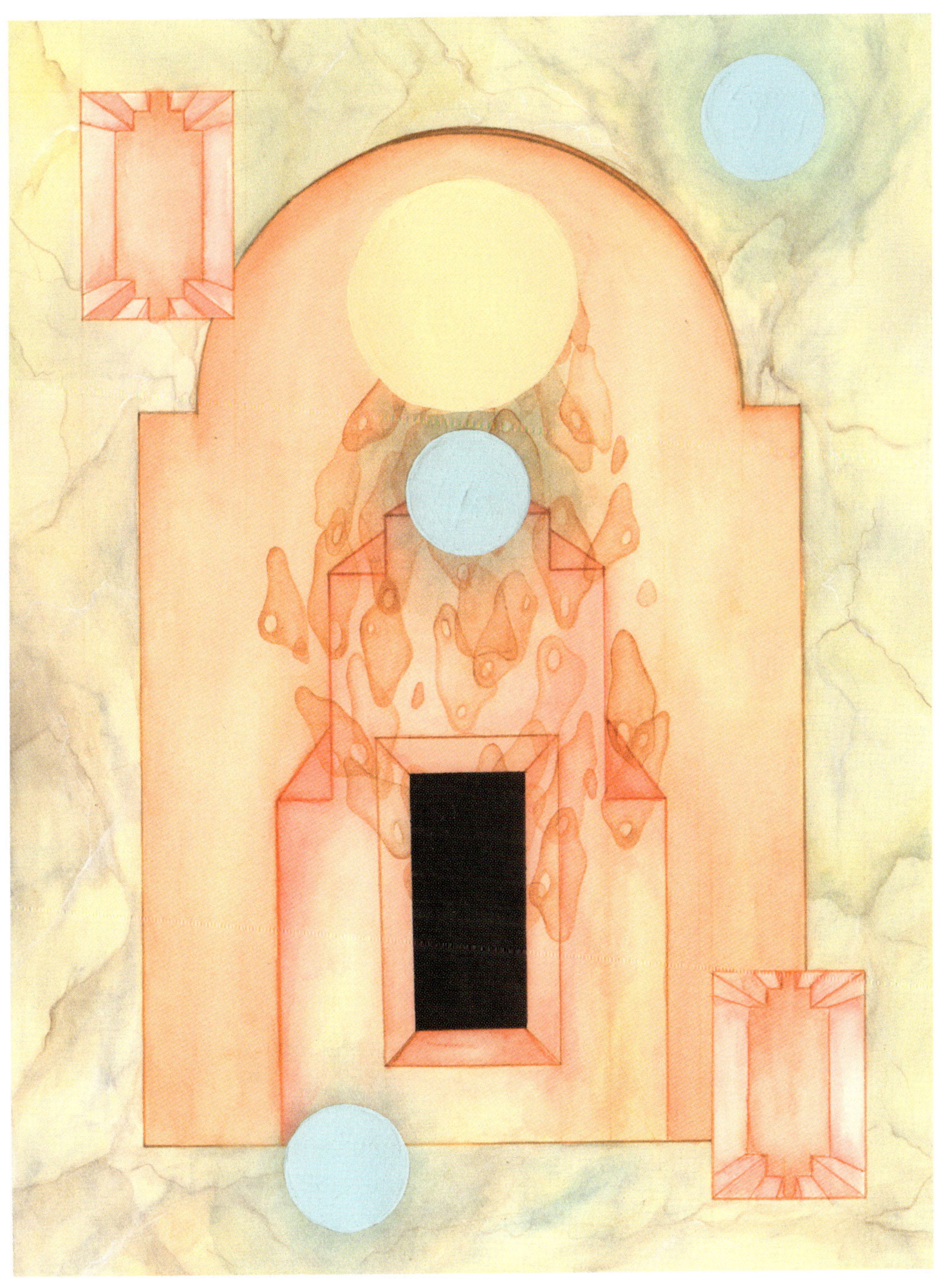

9

This song is a soundwave travelling as long as its molecular collaborators will carry it, where it will end up conserved forever in the museum of unrecoverable vibrations.

Love, an unconstrained love of these energetic fields emanating from a delicate set of processes, hormonal make ups, synapses. A prose-like network of cellular activity and phenomena, subtle mannerisms that provoke so much tenderness and eternal devotion, from one lost coordinate on the temporal plane to another.

You didn't believe me when I told you, the sun is a ghost that haunts the night.

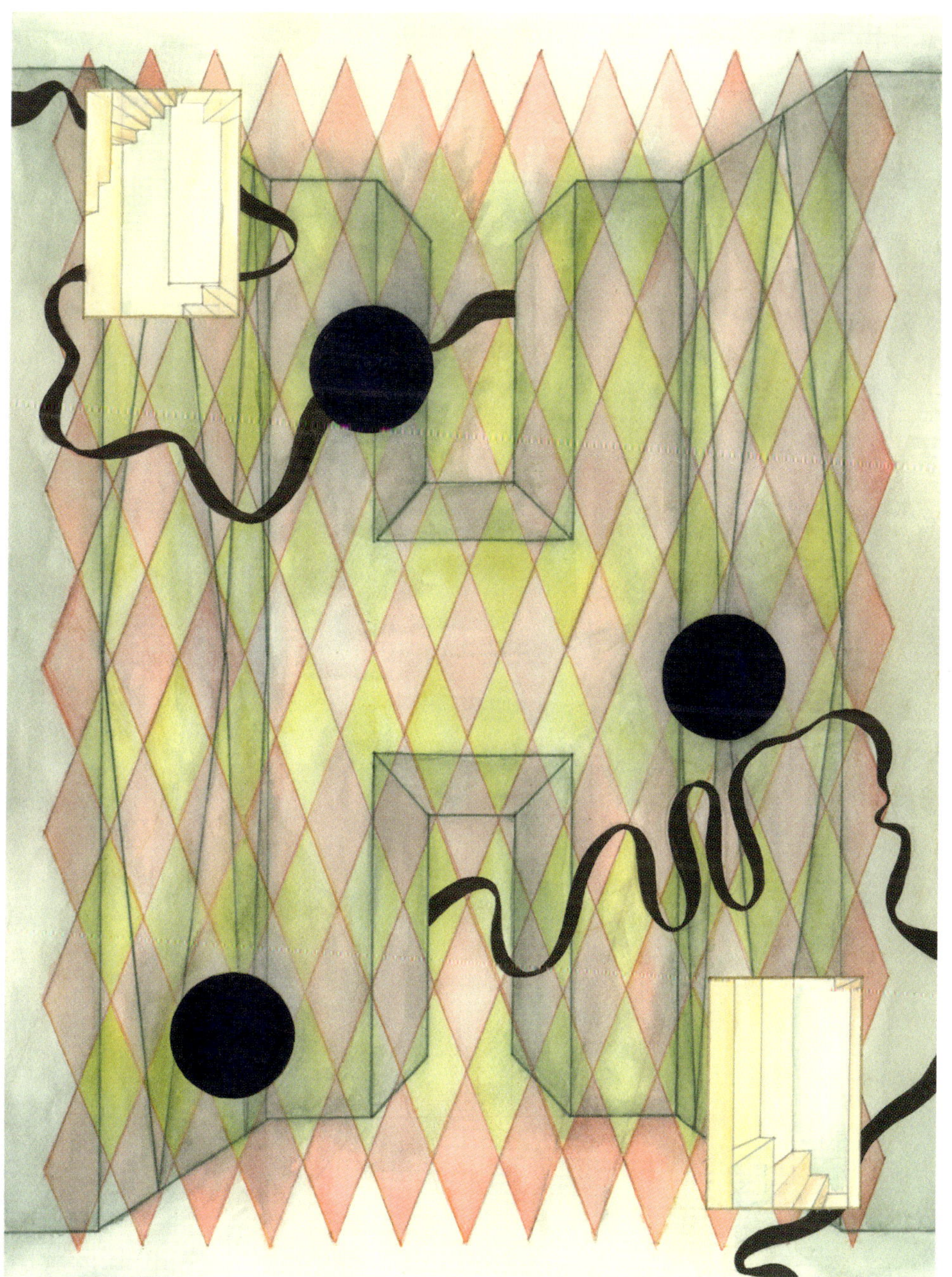

Dissociated Press: An Essay For Tai

Caspar Heinemann

> Here there is continuous intersection of the collapsed Before, After, Below, Above, and behind this a darkness.
>
> It is good to go into the troubled waters of others and to fish in them yourself. For darkness is not only useful to criminals, lovers also know what to do with it. That is why a glance is important which, while it wants and knows progress, also knows it in concealed form or in loops.
>
> - Ernst Bloch, *The Heritage of Our Times*

We see sideways into the room as it really is, hung with hydrangeas and marzipan and a feast of a thousand sideways glances. There is something like a plaque on the wall to karaoke, BDSM, poetry, freely chosen exogenous hormonal systems. Because of the excessively complex lighting design, everything in the room changes colour constantly with the movements of your eyes and feet. This effect is multiplied by the wild abundance of reflective surfaces, tripping the edges of vision over each other. The overall impact is maddening to any attempts to pin down the butterflies, their elegant limbs already splayed across infinite walls (so as to not create the false impression of solidity). There are many oblique folds scattered around the space, superfluous elements and the drama of chiaroscuro forcing you to keep your wits about you. Outside in the wastelands, sans dissenters, everything works properly and everyone agrees the system is entirely sufficient for the task at hand, at least as far as they can tell. The lighting is overhead, as it should be.

Contrary to popular belief, history is a feminised object. Or, more precisely, the practice of history is the masculine imposition of order and logic onto the wild and untamed, and therefore implicitly feminine, object that it itself will come to formulate as history. The practice of history is the sun and the unwieldy events of the past are the moon. "The sun is a ghost that haunts the night" - so begins *The Neon Hieroglyph*, reversing the assumption about who or what is the protagonist, the main event, reminding us of the involuntary status of illumination, questioning the dictate that the object is most itself under the bright lights of the operating table. The cosmology of *The Neon Hieroglyph* draws on the mythology of ergot, and specifically the Italian island of Alicudi, whose inhabitants were said to have tripped continuously for 450 years. The literal truth of this tale is irrelevant, but what it introduces to us is a provocation: what would it be to live in the world from the inside out, in defiance of the alienated outside in of the past 300 years of Western scientific materialism? In this provocation we have the dual elements of being asked to imagine a state of being in a perpetual state of unreality (as understood in a context where psychedelic experience is assumed to be taking a step away from clear perception of reality), and of being challenged by what it means to evoke the story, to take a psychedelic approach to history whereby the cosmological resonance of the tale is respected as its own reality. The Enlightenment told on itself when they called it the Enlightenment, its shaky foundation is the assumption that the light is more real than the dark.

As someone who does and has done less drugs than might be aesthetically assumed, I think often about an expanded understanding of psychedelics, of technologies of the self. This is in no way an original take, more a summation of the flowing back and forth of various 20th century countercultural experimentations, from the dance floor to the dojo to the dungeon. Perhaps a working definition for what I mean by psychedelics is technologies to access altered states of consciousness, although this seems to undermine the reality of what is accessed, so instead we could say, technologies to access additional layers of reality. A formative documentary that I often think about on string theory and particle physics used the metaphor of a fish swimming in a pond, unaware of the world existing above the waterline, entirely believing itself to be experiencing everything possible because of physically lacking the ability to see anything more. Despite its primacy in my cosmology, I can't remember exactly what this was a metaphor for, but the notion stuck with me of there being an entire other world that could be existing simultaneously, even in the same place as our own, that we simply lacked the ability to not only see, but even to conceptualise as existing.

Psychedelics are the technologies that allow us, if not to see above the water line, then at least to experience the sensation of an above. In his unfinished "Introduction to Acid Communism", Mark Fisher argued against the notion that the counterculture of the 1960s contributed to the rise of neoliberalism, countering instead that it was the unwillingness or inability of the left to engage with the weirder, more psychedelic elements of the counterculture that weakened social movements and left these modalities ripe for individualist right-wing appropriation. He goes on to state that to "recall these multiple forms of collectivity is less an act of remembering than of unforgetting, a counter-exorcism of the spectre of a world which could be free." This spectre is what he terms acid communism, referring to both "actual historical developments and to a virtual confluence that has not yet come together in actuality." What Acid Communism, and Fisher's work more generally, pointed to was the danger of positioning the imaginal as politically frivolous, as surplus to the main event of revolution, when in fact there is no revolution without it. Fisher suggested that it is necessary to draw on the past to defeat the crushing present and spirit us into the potential of the future. While it is important to affirm the reality of the historical events he referenced, his crushing it up against a specification of the confluence that has not yet come indicates a desire for a project of "unforgetting" that expands on this. A modest proposal, drawing on what is often felt in psychedelic experience: what would it be to think about history from the perspective of linear time as an illusion? One of the first implications that comes to mind is that not only can we view our small glimpses of liberation as prefiguratively creating a better future, but also as contributing to healing the past. In a psychedelic history, there is no clear line where the past becomes the present becomes the future, and so we are also freed from the teleological premise that the event only ultimately has significance if it was a victory, instead being able to be good in and of itself, regardless of outcome. A psychedelic history would also be necessarily idealist, in both senses, but I mean more controversially, would recognise that our perceptions of past events, real or imagined, carry their own weight, their own performative consequences. Phrased like this, it sounds relatively uncontroversial, but what I mean is they become in some sense literally real. This kind of affective model of relating to history has obvious perils, the clear potential for falling off the cliff into reactionary nostalgia, or failing to listen to the lessons of the past. But that is only one possible story, and ignores the fact that this is already the situation, that there is no neutral alternative, that it is perhaps more experimentally rigorous for the bias to sit on the surface, on the oil wheel of perception. I am aware that all this could be read as exactly the kind of Foucauldian premise that is held as the height of individualism; what I am actually arguing for is a cosmology that promotes a stranger form of collectivity, of recognising our connectedness to a lineage of attempting to grasp the spectre of the world to come. Acknowledging that we have only seen glimpses does not mean we do not want the whole world.

After another night of "sleeping like a medieval person" (my positive, transhistorical reframing of a persistently interrupted sleep pattern), I am left with a half awake image of the lawn of modernism. The lawn of modernism is a municipal fantasy that stretches out from a brutalist housing block, but not the brutal kind, the good old brutalism of 1:1 scale model utopia, hard edges bathed in soft light revealing the truth that on closer inspection there is no hard edge of concrete, more a tentative fraying out of pebbles and sand into the world. The most prominent architectural feature of the lawn of modernism is that the building casts the inverse of a shadow on the lawn, illuminating it not with the harsh securitised glow of floodlight, but an additional serving of daylight on top of the sun, a block of dusty sunlight through dirty glass cast out across the grass on the communal area. There is a total absence of negative space, with the hazardous effect of seeming to endanger the structural reality of the building, threatening it with oblivion at any second, an estate in a constant state of considering whether to walk into the light for the final time.

The closest most of us will get to tripping continuously for years on end is childhood. When I was young, I often experienced an acute sense of haunting at historical sites, best described as the overwhelming embodied knowledge that the past was still happening, exactly where I was, and I just happened to be living in a different channel, living with Toyotas rather than longboats. But if I was to head off on my own, lose my parents and the activity sheets and information boards, I could end up back there. Except not back there, because it all felt more lateral, although even that feels insufficiently non-Euclidean – In Christ There Is No East Or West, etc. This led to an intuitively materialist understanding of history, of circumstance mediating human consciousness. After recovering from being culturally encouraged to think of this as a product of an overactive imagination, my adult beliefs have swollen to accommodate the reality of these experiences, which I now understand as an accurate embodied perception of time, probably accessible to me then as a result of being new to the premise of linearity. My other formative psychedelic childhood experience was with the ability to induce ego death at will, a sensation I now know to be described as dissociation. I remember being around age 7 and staring at the back of the bathroom door, thinking without malice or emotional charge, "This stupid body, this body isn't me" and feeling my sense of selfhood and identity enter soft focus and slip away, rolling my name and the facts of my life around in my mind like they belonged to a stranger. I don't remember how or when I discovered this, and there is no obvious trauma to link it with, but it has stayed with me in varying degrees of intentionality and welcomeness ever since. It was a scary game, much like ghost-hunting, testing myself to see how far I could go into the void, how long I could stay there. I rarely induce it intentionally now, except to check if I still can, but go through phases where it creeps into my everyday, expelling me from the illusion of cohesion. There is an easily pathologised edge to this, but isn't there always, with the divine? As the tripper and the meditator know, there is a paradox whereby the loss of a solid sense of self is often when you feel most yourself, where the disconnection from identity becomes an intense connection with all things, where the edges of yourself blur into all things and yet there is something that remains. This blurring could be politicised as solidarity, the sensation that you have nothing of yourself to lose, and in fact everything to gain, by identification and empathy and synergy across real and imagined spatial and experiential distances.

A Black Box is a system which can be observed with regards to inputs and outputs while its internal workings are entirely obscured, its contents only possible to speculatively deduce based on their effects. Some examples of possible Black Boxes would be algorithms, engines, brains, and I would argue, history. In his elaboration of the concept in *An Introduction to Cybernetics*, W. Ross Ashby uses as evidence of our continuous engagement with Black Boxes in the world the example of a child learning to use a door handle (the input) to control the movement of the door latch (the output), and necessarily doing so without knowledge of the internal workings. He writes that "what is being suggested now is not that Black Boxes behave somewhat like real objects but that the real objects are in fact all Black Boxes, and that we have in fact been operating with Black Boxes all our lives." In *The Cybernetic Brain*, Andrew Pickering unpacks two different approaches to "Black Box ontology". Firstly, the approach of modern science, which is the urge to open the Black Box, the assumption that the path to understanding lies in cognition, transparency, and ultimately representation, exposure of the constituent parts. He contrasts this with a cybernetic approach that posits a performative understanding of the world, a concern with "performance as performance, not as a pale shadow of representation". He argues that cybernetics staged a kind of "ontological theatre" that allowed for a vision of reality characterised by a primacy of reactivity to the present moment, unlimited by modern science's expectation of graspable causality. This focus on performativity gives space for an enchanted, magical engagement with possibility, of listening to the traces of what might be. It is in this spirit that I want to propose that The World Is A Black Box, and a psychedelic worldview (in the expanded sense) is one that recognises the futility of thinking from outside of the box, of attempting to understand the world through examining and representing its contents, because it recognises that there is no outside to the box, no objective tower to cast our searchlights from.

In the manner of a sickly Victorian child taking to bed, I have taken to walking. As in, for my amorphous ills, and with a feverish mix of commitment, resignation, and a dash of opulence. I trawl the suburbs that spider outwards southeasterly from my home in Glasgow, late at night, weeknights only. Walking alone at night as a moment of phenomenological strangeness has persisted in a way that the history haunting hasn't, the blurriness at the edges of the world leading to a perception of everywhere as vertiginously continuous with everywhere else, a stream of associative consciousness where a piece of architectural vernacular takes me back to a moment staring at the side of a building as a child, forgotten for 20 years. There is a teenage wonder in wandering the streets alone at night that has never diminished for me, and as I walk across another street rendered wyrd by the orange glow of still-dominant sodium street lamps I think, this is just like being on drugs! Against all logic, I have always felt safest, most self-possessed, whilst walking alone at night, even whilst nominally a teenage girl, and now a queer-looking (in every sense) man. Aside from the pure luck of having had no experiences to substantially shatter this sensation of safety, I think its origin is the hunch that because the night is not a time of day, the night is outside of space and time, and therefore the daytime order, a situation which could only be of benefit, the daytime order being what it is. Which is not to say there aren't moments — a car drives alongside a little too slowly, a group of teenagers nudge each other. Even when not alone, a man interrupts me talking effusively to my friends about John Cowper Powys to tell us to watch ourselves, reminding us that one can't expect to stand on the streets at night speaking gleefully (limp-wristedly) about notable anarchist pervert novelists without consequences. Homophobes hate jouissance. But these impositions are not about night, they are impositions of daytime order onto the night, the insistence that the way things are usually, normally, should continue to matter now. Although unevenly distributed under current conditions, there is something connective about the fear of the dark, a fear that seems to exceed socialisation, a touch of infinity in the sensation that, everyone has always been scared of this, at least sometimes. This engagement with the nighttime, whether via fear and/or wonder, creates for an attunement to the performative aspects of the world as a physical and psychical space, the absence of the nuts and bolts and specifics giving way to a purely energetic engagement that could be the spirit of place, the place where the known recedes giving way to a source of both fear and liberation. Our perception of the world at night is true in the way that fairytales are true, their excess and embellishment and sparkle pointing to a deeper story, hard to see in the cold hard light of day, when everything is just as it is.

One night after a drink with a friend, still restless, I walk to my local park, with its well-known cruising spot. At no point along the way do I decide to do this, I just observe my feet driving me onwards (the wisdom of dissociation?), until I find myself standing in a loose knot of brambles and rhododendron bushes. I let my eyes adjust and my ears prick up, wait for a flicker of leaf or moonlight. After a few minutes of stumbling the trails to no avail, I open Grindr and Scruff, the harsh glare of my phone sabotaging my pupils' attempts to submit to the night. I'm disappointed to discover that the distance of the nearest people places them firmly outside the park perimeter. The frisson of potential encounter has faded and I am certain I'm on my own. Despite the anticlimactic outcome, I wonder, was it still cruising? Certainly, so then I find myself considering that perhaps I have just had sex, regardless, albeit of an idealistic tenor — the attentiveness, heightened arousal, tentative reciprocation with the perceived actions of an object of desire. There is no line I can comfortably draw around sex that inherently precludes it having been, and so I scramble home oddly satisfied with my encounter in and with the dark.

Like the uncanny dissociative me-not-me effect of seeing yourself outside of the window at night, the shadowy half-self that somehow moves with you, psychedelic technologies set the stage for experiencing the world as it is, not as one expects it to be. I have almost stopped thinking of dissociation as dissociation, as the term seems to imply the primacy of a particular mode of selfhood, that is perhaps in fact one amongst many. Dissociation is what we see when we are destabilised in our sense of what we should be seeing. You see yourself and you are not as you expect to seem. But as the biases of algorithms repeatedly demonstrate, our expectations for the world, including ourselves, are rarely liberating. This is not a question of political perspective, as what you want to happen is not the same as what you expect to happen, and so we are all equally afflicted with the knowledge of our past experiences, of the information we have received about the world. To return to Ashby, in the same chapter on black boxes he writes, "Clearly, 'memory' is not an objective something that a system either does or does not possess; it is a concept that the observer invokes to fill in the gap caused when part of the system is unobservable. The fewer the observable variables, the more will the observer be forced to regard events of the past as playing a part in the system's behaviour." This proposition would suggest that the less knowledge we have of the situation at hand, the more memory required to make sense of it, the less rooted the object becomes in its current time and space. In my model of psychedelic history, I want to argue that the future can also flood in to fill the gap, that we can understand things not just in terms of what has caused them to become what they are, but what what they are says about what they could become. I also relate this to my experiences of dissociation, of becoming an observer to the system of myself, rendered opaque to myself.

As a lifelong dissociative, I often find myself seeking what I've started thinking about as "black box experiences", ones that allow me to think about my own terms of engagement with reality through heightened or altered sensation, that put me in dialogue with the box itself, from the inside out, touching the edges of reality to realise its flimsiness, the insubstantiality of my assumptions about how things should be. In "A Good Drug for A Bad World" (a definitive essay on ketamine and dissociation), P.E. Moskowitz writes about the potential healing powers of psychedelics for depression, their ability to assist you in "rebuilding your brain like a psychedelic architect." However, they ultimately politically conclude, "Ketamine helped me come to terms with my global warming anxiety, but it didn't solve global warming." It should come as no surprise at this point that I don't see this as individual or apolitical, but rather an important crux of political action, essentially establishing a healthy ontological relation to the world, a nourishing cosmology that allows one to continue in the face of overwhelming personal and global suffering. Dissociation, and other psychedelic experiences, allow us to shake our core assumptions about reality and access the mental space where things really could be different, really could be otherwise. Intentional, informed psychedelic experiences can give us the space to see that perhaps consciousness itself is essentially an uninformed, unintentional psychedelic experience. This moment of the zoomed out perspective of dissociation blended with hyperconnectedness invites us to question, with its tenuous reality in and out of mind, what do we want reality to be? While writing this, I looked up Diane di Prima's poem "Rant" with the intention of quoting a single line, only to realise with a combination of amusement and slight dismay that, as is often the case with poetry (that most wholesome of psychedelic technologies), she managed to say in one stanza what I've been attempting to say in 4,000 words:

> history is a living weapon in yr hand
> & you have imagined it, it is thus that you
> "find out for yourself"
> history is the dream of what can be, it is
> the relation between things in a continuum

Acknowledgements

When I consider the duration and spatial dimensions of our world, an incomprehensible almost infinite amount of factors have decided to put us in each other's intimate orbits during this fleeting spectacular apparition of living - little suns in each other's night, knowing love together.

This poem is for you.

STRANGE ATTRACTOR PRESS 2022